# ESSENTIAL DROPS FOR LOVE

# Essential Drops for Love

Kathy Hoppe

&

Connie Bynum

Copyright © 2019 Kathy Hoppe

All rights reserved.

ISBN: 9781711118949

Scriptures taken from the Holy Bible, New International Version®, NIV®. Copyright © 1973, 1978, 1984, 2011 by Biblica, Inc.™ Used by permission of Zondervan. All rights reserved worldwide. www.zondervan.com The "NIV" and "New International Version" are trademarks registered in the United States Patent and Trademark Office by Biblica, Inc.™

# DEDICATION

We would like to dedicate this book to our loving husbands, Jim & Jeff.

# CONTENTS

Preface

Chapter 1    ONCE UPON A TIME    1

Chapter 2    FRIENDSHIP    16

Chapter 3    RESPECT    25

Chapter 4    AFFECTION    35

Chapter 5    TRUST    43

Chapter 6    INTIMACY    52

Chapter 7    COMMITMENT    59

Chapter 8    COMMUNICATION    68

Chapter 9    FORGIVENESS    77

Chapter 10    HAPPILY, AFTER ALL    86

Resources Cited    95

About the Authors    107

Endnotes    109

# PREFACE

As we envisioned our series, *Essential Drops*, we wanted to create an experience with essential oils that touched every part of our lives. It made sense to begin with *Essential Drops for Living* wherein the focus is upon our inner lives and aligning that with our outer world. The following step that seemed most natural was to move to our love lives, especially with our significant others. That's how this second book in the series arose, *Essential Drops for Love.*

We think we have some things to share with you about love relationships. Connie and her husband, Jim, have been married for 43 years. Kathy and Jeff Hoppe have been married for 38 years. One cannot be a couple for that length of time without experiencing the usual ups and downs in relationships, the crises of life, raising children, moving across the country numerous times, facing temptations, having conflict, and, in the end, continuing to remain committed to the same partner. Even more important is that both couples are in love!

We want you to have successful relationships that are healthy and bring life to you and your partner. We believe this can happen. So, we bring our individual experiences and expertise to you once again. Connie's knowledge of health, happiness, healing, and essential oils informs us on the level of practical application. Kathy's experience as a marriage therapist and understanding of problems and successes of couples guide us in offering sound advice for relationships.

Our first book, *Essential Drops for Living,* was designed to be primarily inspirational. We decided to approach love differently. In *Essential Drops for Love,* we hope you find it inspiring. Still, more than that, we want to inform you what it takes to have the type of love that lasts forever while offering some ways that you can use essential oils to enhance the characteristics needed to strengthen your bond.

As in our previous book, you'll notice that we use the singular pronoun. This makes the text readable, although our experiences are unique. Unless otherwise noted, all scriptures are from the New International Version of the Bible.

All oils mentioned in this guide are Young Living essential oils. If you desire to become a customer, then you can access those at our website: https://www.beyondbelief.life/young-living. Please take a few minutes daily to enjoy your journey through this guide. Let us know how your relationships change for better!

*Kathy & Connie*

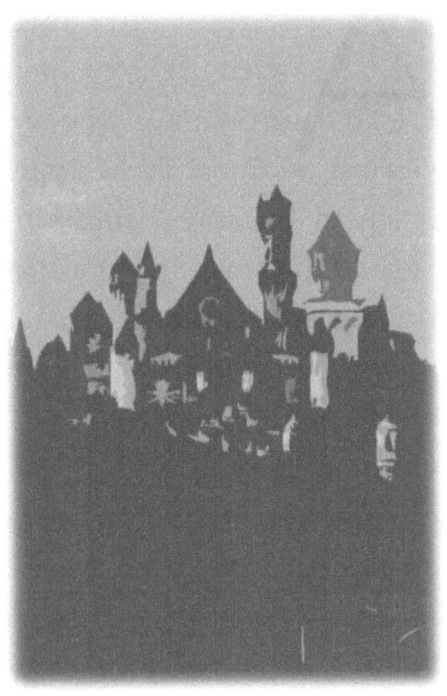

## Chapter 1
# ONCE UPON A TIME

*Once upon a time is now.*

Emilie Autumn

All good fairy tales begin the same way with *"Once upon a time."* This start informs the listener something exciting is about to happen. I recall how thrilled my child became when I used that phrase, even if I was making up a bedtime story about him. It increases a sense of anticipation as the hearer knows there will be a good guy, a bad guy, a damsel or don in distress, a fight, and the right person will win, and all will be well. Even I get goosebumps when reading an engaging tale. Sometimes I'm so enthused about the novel I'm reading I'll skip to the end to read the final pages. I still read the "in-between" stuff because there's no drama without it.

But what about "real life" love stories? Sometimes people try to cast away or deny the in-between struggle to get straight to the end. We meet, fall in love, and live happily ever after, right? That's how it should be. Or is it? I remember a couple coming for marriage counseling. They were married for less than a year. The husband said, "I didn't know marriage would be so hard." I replied, "Marriage with the wrong person is hell. Marriage to the right person is a lot of hard work."

I'm a realist, and often disappoint my clients when I tell them what they face. I hate deflating their balloon of happy expectations. Yet I know if they keep trying to float the bubble high, they will face some unforeseeable force which will blow it somewhere they don't desire to be. Or some event will unexpectedly prick the bright ball and with one big POP! their dream will disappear as quickly as it arrived. Beginning with "Once upon a time" is nice. But the in-between is vital to the relationship.

Joseph Campbell outlined a structure for good fiction called "The Hero's Journey." The story line begins in an ordinary world and moves into a situation where the hero faces a test. He or she overcomes an evil force, a terrible event, or resolves a difficult dilemma, and returns to normal life.[1] The protagonist spends at least half the time in the middle of the drama, the in-between, because this is where we can see the hero's real character.[2] So, it is with us in living. Our real nature is only plain when we face life's ugly moments.

When we first meet someone and fall in love, we don't see them accurately. We're using our best behaviors just as they are. You've heard the quote, "love is blind." It turns out it's true, but for reasons you may not know. During the initial attraction to another person, our bodies release higher levels of oxytocin, the "feel-good" hormone, which alters our perceptions of the other person. It's like wearing "rose-colored glasses."[3] High levels of oxytocin will remain for at least six to nine months before decreasing.[4] Oxytocin enhances relationships by increasing trust, empathy, fidelity, and bonding.[5] But what happens when the love hormone falls back to normal, and the rose glasses fall off?

Whether time or an event or difficulty arises, couples will face every day living with one another, with all the bodily functions, irritable habits, and angry words. This is when the real testing begins. The in-between is now at play, and couples will spend most of their lives together in this twilight zone. This will not be a fairy tale. But it will be the period in which the potential for long-lasting love develops. It is during this phase you can move from a "feel good," temporary hook-up to a lasting and satisfying love connection.

Some may wonder why longer relationships are

better when moving on to a new one can raise oxytocin again. It's a lot of work to keep love alive! Lasting and strong relationships are healthy for everyone. They increase resiliency, improve one's sense of well-being, increase life expectancy, improve career achievement, and decrease financial problems.[6] If we can make our partnerships in love remain, many more of us will be happier people.

There is research on creating oxytocin delivery via nose sprays.[7] I can see the commercials now. Shot opens with man frowning at his wife. "Irritated with your wife? One sniff will restore your interest in her." The husband turns away, uses nasal spray, and turns back to his wife smiling. The camera pans to a woman lying in bed, and her husband reaches out to her. She groans in dismay at the thought of his request but reaches for her nasal spray and sniffs. Turning towards her husband, she smiles and says, "How can I make you happy today?" The husband grins. Hmm. Are you ready for a nasal spray? I can't wait to read the ingredient label.

The problem with this notion is it presumes we can maintain the initial infatuation that begins a relationship. Is this what we want or need? Let's think back to our hero's journey again, and the in-between. The character-revealing, middle-of-the-story, facing dilemmas part of life becomes both endearing and enduring. Irreplaceable bonds form during this time. It provides the grit in a couples' life that strengthens commitment and love.

When people lose the emotional appeal and must deal with the drama of life, they become discouraged, disheartened, or disillusioned, and that's when they choose to "hang it up." If a couple has a lot of outward conflicts, they most likely will separate within the first seven years of marriage. However, if they're on a "slow burn" marriage, and the disappointment and disagreement remain subterranean, they can make it up to 16 years.[8] Whatever the case, couples wait an average of six years before they even seek help,[9] and it may be too late.

We want to help you before you reach the end of the relationship. If you understand what it takes to make it through the boring, the tough, the best, and the difficult times, and you face those challenges head-on and well-equipped, you can have a satisfying life with your partner. That is the purpose of this book.

Through our experiences in living and loving, in health and wellness studies, in marriage counseling and teaching, we've identified some critical characteristics for you to focus on and develop further. Those qualities that make a relationship last include *friendship, respect, affection, trust, intimacy, commitment, positivity, communication, and forgiveness.* We've dedicated a chapter to each of these qualities and provide you with information, inspiration, advice, essential oils, and activities to strengthen these in your love life. Some of these chapters will ask for reflection alone, while others will request you engage your loved one in conversation or participation in an exercise. All will lead you to a deeper and more durable connection to your partner.

This guide can help you in your current or future relationships. However, some of you may already be in a troubling spot with your lover and are uncertain if you can remain. If this is true, we ask you seek help from a licensed professional counselor or marriage and family therapist. This book is not a substitute for therapy, nor will it help if you've waited too long, or there are too many existing issues. Likewise, some situations call for extensive help. If you are in an abusive interchange (emotional, physical, or sexual), or if either partner is engaged in substance abuse or misuse, we request you seek professional help. **Stop, put this book down, and call someone for help.** This guide cannot repair a relationship in which there is a significant danger, ongoing abuse, denial of problems, or active substance use.

Those pairs who will receive the most benefit from this guide are stable relationships in which some or most of the characteristics we've identified are already present but need further care or development. If you have most of these, we believe this book can help you, and we encourage you to proceed.

## SPIRITUAL REFLECTION

*The Lord God said, "It is not good for the man to be alone. I will make a helper suitable for him." . . . But for Adam no suitable helper was found. So the Lord God caused the man to fall into a deep sleep; and while he was sleeping, he took one of the man's ribs and then closed up the place with flesh. Then the*

*Lord God made a woman from the rib he had taken out of the man, and he brought her to the man. The man said, "This is now bone of my bones and flesh of my flesh; she shall be called 'woman,' for she was taken out of man.*

Genesis 2:18 – 37

In reading the creation story, we hear the plan for partnership. The Divine One sees that the first human needed another being and so he creates a mate for him. The key focus is on the need for relationship. "It is not good for the man to be alone." Most of us have a desire to share life with someone.

Our problem becomes looking for the "perfect" person. Of course, he or she doesn't exist. Yet there are people who are more suitable. Notice how the scripture remarks on this. "But for Adam no suitable helper was found." It makes us wonder if a search happened. Was God looking elsewhere or was the man? The best partner was one who suited the man and allowed both to become one flesh. This unity is an important concept.

In looking for a lover, it's vital to find someone with whom we can unite, share the journey, and have the same mind. It is that harmony that weaves us together in perfect song. God's desire is that we experience relationship, so we do not face life alone. It doesn't mean we have something magical, but we can have partnerships that bring joy and fulfillment in our lives.

Think about your current loved one. Do you remember what first attracted you to him or her? What quality or characteristic captured your attention? You chose this person, not another one, for some reason. Reflect on how that individual made you feel alive. And you did the same for him or her. There was something in those first few days or months that pulled you together.

I remember meeting my husband at a wedding. The following Sunday he asked me to take him to the airport. I felt like I was losing a part of myself. That's when I knew I had something special.

What about when you fell in love with your partner? You could have chosen anyone, but you didn't. Were you foolish? Were you blind? Perhaps you were not. There was something that brought you together. It's time to rediscover that.

## Essential Oil: Myrrh

Since you're beginning this journey in your relationship, you need emotional balance. We want you to be free of stress and worry. We suggest you use some myrrh, which can bring spiritual awareness and emotional insight to your relationship.[10] Inhale some myrrh and complete the following action.

# TAKE ACTION

It's time to assess your relationship. We've developed a short assessment to help. Answer the questions and score the quiz. See how your relationship is doing. There is no research on this questionnaire, and it is not indicative of impending relationship failure. It will help you think about the qualities of a healthy relationship.

**Essential Drops for Love Questionnaire**

Answer each item below using the following rating scale:
1 = poor or none
2 = a little
3 = sometimes
4 = most of the time
5 = almost always

| Ex. Rating | Question |
|---|---|
| 3 | I always show my partner respect. |
|  | I view my partner as a good friend. |

| | |
|---|---|
| | My partner forgives me easily. |
| | I am affectionate with my partner. |
| | We talk through decisions carefully. |
| | I ask my partner for his or her opinion on things. |
| | There are things my partner knows & keeps secret about me. |
| | We both agree on the frequency & type of sex we enjoy together. |
| | I do not take things personally when my partner says things. |
| | My partner does not take things personally that I say. |
| | There are things my partner has told me that I keep secret. |
| | We have a quality sex life. |
| | I treat my partner like a good friend. |
| | We can agree to disagree on |

|   |   |
|---|---|
|   | certain topics. |
|   | I can envision the future with my partner. |
|   | My partner asks for my opinions on things. |
|   | I forgive my partner easily. |
|   | My partner is affectionate with me. |
|   | We have similar dreams for the future. |

*Total your score. Scoring:*

41 – 50    Your relationship needs work.

51 – 60    You may need marital counseling.

61 – 70    You have some areas of growth.

71 – 80    Good job. Need more help?

81 – 90    Congratulations! You're doing well.

# REFLECT

What's one thing you learned about relationships from this chapter? Did it surprise you? How does this chapter help you in your current relationship? What do you need to do to make your relationship healthier?

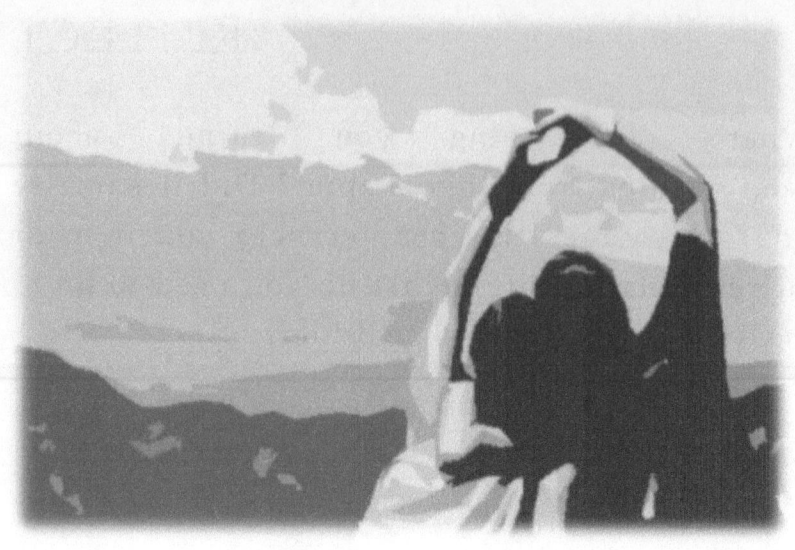

# Chapter 2
# FRIENDSHIP

*You are my best friend as well as my lover, and I do not know which side of you I enjoy the most. I treasure each side, just as I have treasured our life together.*

Nicholas Sparks

Recently I noticed an article stated, "Your wife is not your best friend. Don't confuse marriage and friendship." As I read the article, I tried to make sense of the advice. Still it didn't add up. The author of the article is quoting research from the field of economics. The related study is about individual happiness, financial matters, and has little to do with overall couple satisfaction.

It's disappointing to see articles which lead us in the opposite direction from 40 years of couple research. John Gottman and Julie Schwarz Gottman are leading researchers of relationships. In 1986, John Gottman and Robert Levenson set up "The Love Lab" and determined the couples who were "masters" and those who were "disasters." There isn't room here to discuss these studies. There is evidence that friendship in marriage separates successful and unsuccessful couples.[11] Thus, it makes sense to build marital friendship.

So, what does friendship entail? *The Stanford Encyclopedia of Philosophy* states friendship involves the care and concern for another and has the other person's best interest in mind and includes intimacy.[12] In Greek philosophy, this love is *philia*, meaning love for another based on what the other person needs.[13] This is what the scripture says in John 15:13, "Greater love has no one than this: to lay down one's life for one's friends."

If I want to forsake my life for a friend, I must be familiar with this person inside and out. I need to understand what motivates them, what pleases them, their best triumphs, and their most significant struggles. It means I respect and admire this person, and, most likely, receive those in return. Seal and colleagues say it means not judging the other but listening to provide a helpful perspective.[14]

To be friends with my lover means being playful with him or her in the little and big things. It involves making time for my partner and ensuring they feel important and acknowledged.[15] If my lover is my friend, I will show a genuine interest in what they think is necessary and I will be the best ally my partner can have.[16]

However, friendships need attention and time. McKenna says this love–friendship focuses on knowing and understanding one's partner while building fondness and admiration, and appreciating the small, routine tasks which engage each daily.[17]

Does this describe what you have? It requires you know your partner on many levels. You take time when you see this person to inquire about their day, their stresses, their challenges, hopes, and dreams. It means you greet the person, look them in the eye, and you try to understand their point of view in conversations. You treat them with respect and kindness. You ask yourself, "Is this how I would treat my best friend?" If the answer is no, then you need to re-assess your view of this person.

Often, I hear individuals place responsibility (and blame) on their partner. Here's what I want you to know: **your relationship will not improve until you decide you have ownership of the problem.** Your job is to keep this relationship alive! How do you keep your plants alive? You water them, you give them the proper light, you tend to them, you prune them, you feed them. Are you providing your partner with the same care you give your plants? Given the right amount of attention, your plant will continue to grow.

Do you want your spouse to be more engaging? Talk about your lover's interests. Do you want your partner to be more loving? Be kind. Do you want your lover to be gentler? Speak in a softer tone of voice. Be the friend to your partner you desire him or her to be to you. They may, or may not, reciprocate, but you will not know if they can be your friend if you do not act as a friend first.

I realize these may be difficult words for you to hear if you are struggling in your relationship. I'm so sorry if you do not have a friend in your partner. The question becomes both can you become friends, and how can you do so? I want to offer you hope. When you offer admiration and fondness, focusing on the positive aspects, personality traits, and things your lover does well, you find your view of him or her changes.

# Spiritual Reflection

*His mouth is sweetness itself; he is altogether lovely. This is my beloved, this is my friend, daughters of Jerusalem.*

Song of Songs 5:16

This is such an interesting verse. It's hard to find anywhere else in scripture where lovers are called friends. Some might argue that this verse is only talking about friendship. But if one reads the entire chapter here, it's pretty clearly love. The passage says the following: "my heart began to pound for him," and "my heart sank at his departure." That's not something I would say about my friend. But it is what I might think about someone with whom I'm in love.

How wonderful it is to think that you can be both a lover and a friend. Bruce Lee wrote, "Love is like a friendship caught on fire. In the beginning a flame, very pretty, often hot and fierce, but still only light and flickering. As love grows older, our hearts mature and our love becomes as coals, deep-burning and unquenchable."[18]

Isn't this what we desire? To have companionship and love? Yet, the question you must consider is whether you treat your partner as if he or she is your best friend. How does that change your view of him or her? What sorts of things must you do to show friendship towards your loved one?

In my relationship with my spouse, I do things for him that he enjoys. One day I remember planting bulbs in the garden. I don't like gardening, but someone gave me these tulips and I felt an obligation to plant them. My spouse was also working outside. When we started indoors a few hours later, he said, "This is the best time I've ever had with you." I thought, "Huh. I didn't even realize how meaningful this was for him." I stored that in my heart to remind myself being friends and lovers means I grow our relationship by doing something he enjoys, even if it means I don't enjoy it. That's what friends do for one another.

# Essential Oil: Ylang Ylang

Ylang ylang is ideal in providing balance in one's personality. It reduces frustration and harsh judgment.[19] It creates a sense of peace and can lessen any anger while helping to release fears.[20] Zeck explains ylang ylang will help you become more conscious of how you affect others while deepening your relationships.[21] You can use ylang ylang in your bath or in a diffuser. Use the following activities to build friendship.

# Take Action

Choose 3-4 of the following activities to do with your partner. Try them on just like you do clothing, some will work sometimes, others will work better at other times.

1. Choose a time each week to spend time with your partner. Allow nothing to interfere with this time.

2. Take turns exploring your interests. If he enjoys sports events, attend those. If she enjoys artistic endeavors, go to a painting

class with her.

3. Develop a set of questions you can carry to dinner out. Make some topics fun and some more serious.

4. Set some goals together. What is something you would like to accomplish this year that includes both of you?

# REFLECT

In what ways is my partner my friend? What do I admire most about my partner? What can my partner do to help our friendship? Have I told him/her this?

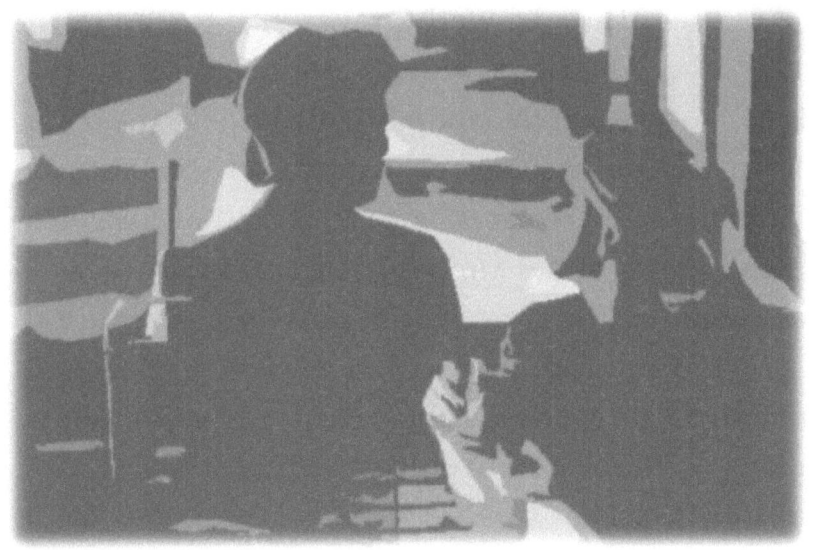

Chapter 3
# RESPECT

*Respect flows two ways and can mean as much to the giver as to the one receiving.*

David Anthony Durham

Gallup is well-known for its polls of American values. In April 1981, the research company provided the first World Values Survey, repeated that same study in 1990, and performed a partial update in 2007. When asking about the most important values in marriage, adults in all three polls placed mutual respect at the top. In the 1981 poll, it was second only to faithfulness with 91% of all respondents noting the importance of respect in relationships.[22]

There is little research on respect in relationships; most likely people assume that respect is already a valued commodity among couples. But, in studies of abusive relationships, respect is absent from those relationships.[23] Your behaviors, tone of voice, and demeanor matter and can undermine your relationship. It's also known as contempt.[24] This makes respect a valuable characteristic of healthy relationships.

What does it mean to respect your partner? It is an attitude, being caring and supportive, and distributing power, honoring and valuing the other person's beliefs, opinions, and personality.[25] It's foundational for romantic relationships. The degree to which couples offer respect relates to relationship satisfaction and commitment.[26] It encompasses paying attention, showing curiosity towards your partner, creating an open dialogue, empowering your loved one, offering healing, and practicing self-respect.[27]

When you respect another individual, you withhold judgment. Instead, you listen, allowing the person to state their thoughts. You hear them out without defending your own position or offering a rebuttal. You accept the other person's point of view as valid, even when you disagree with it.[28]

If we start at the level of basic human rights, most of us will agree all humans receive dignity and respect. That's the moral position. It means allowing people the freedom to express themselves.[29] But respect goes even further in a committed relationship. It means being willing to accept influence from the other person.[30]

How does respect develop in partnerships? The first key is mutuality. It means understanding that there is a power balance in all relationships. Power is not a problem when respect is present.

Respect is sensitive to attitudes, and thus can go up or down in couples, depending on the respect offered. To get respect, one must first give respect. That's called reciprocity.[31]

Having respect for your partner also means that you will honor and protect the personal boundaries of that person and accepting that those may differ from your own. It means being aware that you are different from your loved one, and that you are accepting of those dissimilarities.[32]

Respect begins with you as you show your support of your partner by building them up, speaking positively about them to others, and realizing that your loved one is an imperfect person. Just as you are also flawed. You overlook those defects in the other because of your love and respect for them.[33] Treating your partner with honor means you focus on what's right instead of what's wrong with them.

What can you do to show respect to your significant other? Behaviors speak loudly. Pay attention to your posture and facial expressions. Rolling your eyes is a universal sign of contempt so it's important to remain cognizant of your eye contact. Your tone of voice shows your level of respect. Speak gently but firmly when needed. Do small acts of kindness for your partner. Offer to do a task you wouldn't normally do that benefits your lover.

Talk with him or her about personal boundaries. My spouse does not like me to talk about him in public or with others or tell others what he may or may not do. I try to honor that. I'm more open and willing to let my spouse speak about me to others or tell them how I think. But knowing those variances and then being mindful of those boundaries strengthens the relationship. Be thankful. I know it's important to express my gratitude to my husband, and I must remind myself to be grateful for his presence and influence in my life.

## Spiritual Reflection

*Submit to one another out of reverence for Christ . . . For this reason a man will leave his father and mother and be united to his wife, and the two will become one flesh. This is a profound mystery—but I am talking about Christ and the church. However, each one of you also must love his wife as he loves himself, and the wife must respect her husband.*

Ephesians 5:21, 31–33.

Paul is often miscategorized as misogynous by people. To do so is to misunderstand the apostle. He's actually an advocate for women, stating "There is no male or female" in Galatians 3:28 and speaking of Phoebe as deaconess in Romans 16. There are other instances of his support of women, but it is this passage in Ephesians, which is misinterpreted most frequently.

Notice how Paul first commends that both partners should submit to one another. What does that mean? Submission is an act of giving or offering something to another person out of respect. It confers power to another person in recognition of the other's trustworthiness. If my friend says, "Trust me. I know where to send you for help," I do so. If my friendship is solid, and my experiences are honest, then I have no reason to distrust my comrade. I am yielding control of something to them.

We tend to resist this notion of submission as if it's a bad thing to do. There are times, however, when it's better. We do it all the time. It happens when our teachers determine our grade, or when our bosses redefine our job, or our kids tell us when to pick them up. Those are acts of giving, of submission to someone's will. It's respectful.

So why wouldn't we want to respect our best friend and lover? If he, as Paul states, loves me as much as his own body, then I have no worries. He will take care of me as if he's taking care of his physical being. But, we're one flesh, right? So, that also means he yields to me at times. He readily receives my influence. A key characteristic of happily married couples is when the husband readily receives influence from his wife.[34] That's what it means to be one, but it can only happen in relationships where there is mutual respect.

Please hear me. Earlier in this book, I mentioned how this is intended for partners who have one another's best interests in mind, who love and support one another. I do not expect that you offer yourself if those do not exist in your love life. The idea of mutuality is key. You give freely, even as your loved one gives to you. If that is not occurring, then something is wrong, and you cannot proceed until something changes.

Respect comes easy when one is treated with reverence. Indeed, it becomes a joy to offer deference in that moment because I know it will return to me.

# Essential Oil: Melissa

To build respect, you must let go of resentment and the need for power in a relationship. Often, the hurt feelings you encounter over time are because of repeated failures in your relationship and hardens your heart. Respect cannot develop in a closed heart. Melissa becomes an excellent choice to use. "Like a beam of light on a dark winter's day, Melissa softens extreme emotions, eases resentment, gladdens the heart and engages the soul in its own graceful rhythm."[35]

Melissa comes from the *Melissa officinalis*.[36] Davis[37] states that Melissa can expand your feelings of love. It can strengthen your love response, leading to the expression of hurt and anger.[38] It also soothes resentment, allowing you to reflect and be thankful.[39]

## TAKE ACTION

Here are some ways to generate respect in your relationship.

*Activity 1: Speaking Gently*

Practice responding in a gentle manner. How does speaking softly to your partner alter your interactions? Try this when you need to bring up a sensitive issue. Ask if it's a good time to talk. Then proceed cautiously.

*Activity 2: Listening Actively*

When your partner talks with you, empty your mind. Your goal is to understand. Respond by stating the most important issue. Ask if they feel understood. If no, try again. Then check with them. If they still don't feed understood, ask how they will know when you understand. What will you do or say differently?

# Reflect

In what ways do you show respect for your partner? How does your partner respect you?

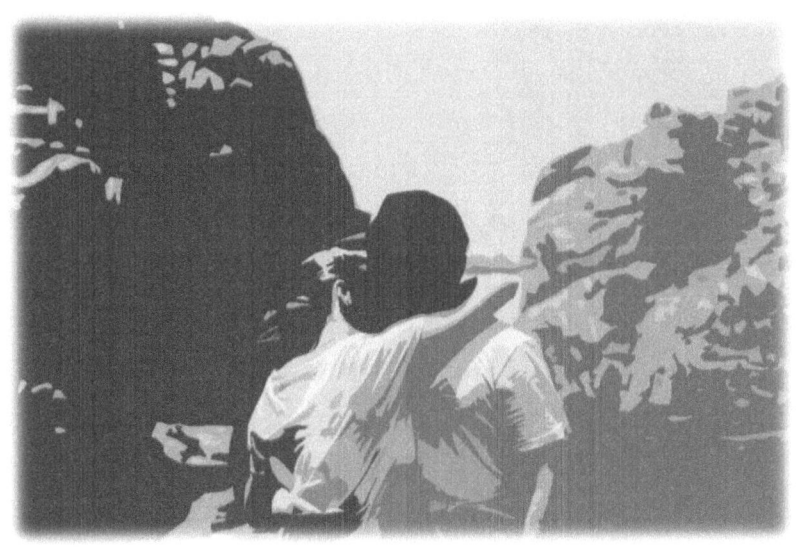

Chapter 4
# AFFECTION

*Hugging:
the truest form of giving and receiving.*

Carol 'CC' Miller

Kissing. It's so much fun! I love doing research on kissing. Here's what I learned. A French kiss can use up to 29 facial muscles. A kiss contains up to 278 bacteria (95% are non-dangerous), can quicken your pulse up to 100 beats a minute, and burns up to 3 calories per kiss.[40] The longest-lasting kiss happened in Pattaya, Thailand, on February 12-14, 2013, and lasted for 58 hours, 35 minutes, and 58 seconds.[41] Whew, that's a long time. Could you do that?

So why is affection crucial in a relationship, anyway? Physical love is essential for your health and for your lover. Did you know that physical affection improves your mental health, your physical well-being, academic performance, and decreases depression and loneliness?[42] Increased kissing over six weeks can reduce your total cholesterol and decrease your perceived stress.[43] Sign me up!

What happens with physical affection? Remember that "cuddle hormone," oxytocin? Whenever we receive or give hugs, our bodies release more of the hormone. Higher levels of oxytocin make us feel closer to the person we're hugging, even if the relationship isn't perfect.[44] Oxytocin helps us feel happier with our partners. Affectionate people also have higher self-esteem and better mental health. They are more likely to be in long-term romantic relationships.[45]

So, does this mean you have to kiss more? Maybe. But other types of physical affection are as important. There are seven types of physical affection: holding hands, back rubs/massages, caressing/stroking, cuddling/holding, kissing on the lips, and kissing on the face.[46] Of these, massages are the most selfless, while caressing or stroking is least important to relationship satisfaction.[47] Other interesting information is that cuddling, hugging, and kissing on the lips predict how easily a couple will resolve conflicts.[48] More hugging for me, please!

Many studies show that relationship satisfaction and physical affection are connected.[49] There is a theory called the Affection Exchange Theory that states a person's need for physical touch is a built-in drive that helps people form significant relationships.[50]

Think about that first kiss. I remember mine so well. I was 14 years old (don't tell my momma this) and was on the dance floor with a guy from my school choir. His name was Paul, and he didn't ask me to *go to* the dance, but he asked me *to dance* with him when I arrived. And then, before I knew it, he kissed me! WOW! Excitedly, I fell in love with Paul right away. Our relationship probably lasted less than a few months, but the memory of that first kiss remains alive.

As I mentioned, kissing isn't the only form of affection. Nowadays, I love to sit and hold hands or have my back rubbed or massaged by my spouse. And I feel closer to him when he does it. Now I see that it keeps us healthier. So, more please! Let's show the world how to be more physically affectionate.

# Spiritual Reflection

**HE:** *Your cheeks are beautiful with earrings, your neck with strings of jewels. We will make you earrings of gold, studded with silver.*

**SHE:** *My beloved is to me a sachet of myrrh resting between my breasts.*

**HE:** *How beautiful you are, my darling! Oh, how beautiful! Your eyes are doves.*

**SHE:** *How handsome you are, my beloved! Oh, how charming! And our bed is verdant.*

**HE:** *The beams of our house are cedars; our rafters are firs.*

Song of Songs 1:10, 13, 15–17


What a fun scene! Who knew the Bible could be sexy? Yet, in this scenario we witness the playfulness and teasing between two lovers. It's an affectionate display of romance. It's this type of warmth we need in our relationships. I can almost picture the couple chasing and hiding from one another behind the cedars, and then peeking out to discover each other.

How often do you experience this in your love life? Life brings such busy schedules that we forget playfulness is part of affection. It's the hide and seek that preps us for the serious lovemaking. It's necessary for long-lasting relationships that lose their spark.

I remember such a moment. We were at a motel for a soccer tournament. I was standing on the balcony and I saw a man come walking across the courtyard. I thought, "Wow. What a handsome guy!" I giggled and he looked up. Then I tried to hide but he found me. I blushed and he smiled. He was my husband. In that moment, we re-captured the essence of affectionate play.

This interaction occurs when you are open and curious. It occurs in times when you see your lover through new eyes and are thankful for him or her. It's in the flirting and being present in the moment that brings freshness in your encounters. As you open yourself to experience your partner in new ways, you discover things you normally overlook. Allow those times to increase your desire for your partner.

## Essential Oil: Cinnamon Bark

Need a little help? Sometimes we get accustomed to one another and forget that touching is so important. To help increase your desire, try some cinnamon bark. It serves as a libido enhancer and creates warm and fond memories. Cinnamon bark also awakens your inner self to the present moment and leaves you open to experiences.[51] It can help with self-confidence, sexual expression, and clearing trapped emotions. Place a few drops of cinnamon bark in the bedroom, or add to a glass spray bottle and spritz the sheets. However, be careful with the amount because skin can be sensitive to it. Diluting with a carrier oil before direct application helps.[52]

## TAKE ACTION

Try a few of these things this week:

1. Next time you kiss your spouse or partner, hold the kiss for at least six seconds.

2. Offer a back massage. It's a selfless act that will help both of you feel closer.

3. Talk with your spouse or partner about the seven types of physical affection. You can make this a fun guessing game.

4. Hold hands in public or while watching a movie.

5. Practice other forms of affection. Surprise your spouse.

## REFLECT

What prevents you from offering physical affection to your partner? What type of physical affection makes you feel closer to your partner?

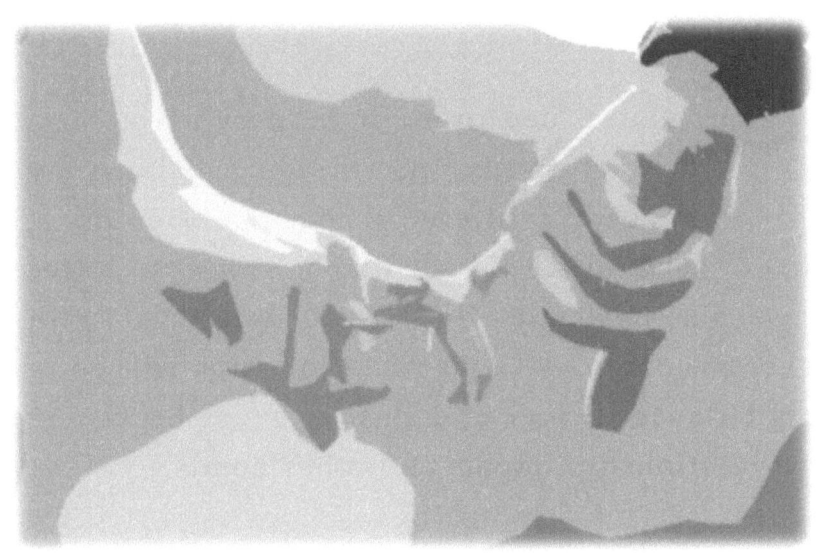

# Chapter 5
# TRUST

*The best way to find out if you can trust somebody is to trust them.*

Ernest Hemingway

She turned to me with teary eyes. "You must think I'm stupid." Shaking my head, I offered a tissue. "He did it again," she cried. Most likely she will never trust her husband. He's been unfaithful with several women. All other relationships will be in this balance of fear and desire. Trust broken in one relationship impacts all other bonds.

The couple qualities in this book are interdependent. It's not possible for two people to love without trust. Hemingway is correct. One cannot have trust unless one is vulnerable. Like respect, trust goes both ways and builds on mutuality. When you have an opportunity to betray your lover, and you don't, you build confidence. Likewise, confronted with a chance to hurt you and he doesn't, fidelity increases.[53]

What is trust? According to research, there are two types: calculus-based trust (CBT) and identification-based trust (IBT). I know, confusing right? We use CBT every day and in all interactions. It builds one step at a time, as people prove themselves trustworthy. It rises when someone has consistent behavior and keeps his or her promises.[54] IBT is more personal and related to one's emotions. Shared values, and a unified outlook on life increases IBT. Lovers develop this as they get to know one another and discover connection, motivations, and goals. It requires a high emotional investment, and if cracked, is difficult to repair.[55]

Belief is integral for healthy functioning. Feeling safe, being open, and willing to offer vulnerability despite the risks of being hurt define trust.[56] Trust is a powerful predictor of relationship success. "Do I think my partner will have my back when I need it?" "Will my lover cheat on me?" "Does he keep his promises?" "If I fail at something, will she support me?" Dependability is vital. If I'm uncertain about any of my questions, I will become more sensitive to all that my lover says and does.[57]

Authenticity proves trustworthiness.[58] People who are authentic are the most faithful partners because they are sensitive to their lovers and they are unable or unwilling to hide feelings.[59] Moral integrity is a key motivator for authenticity, although some people may become truthful to a fault and learn not all thoughts and feelings help a relationship.[60] Some things are best kept to oneself.

In his book, *The Science of Trust,* John Gottman says that trust increases resiliency in couples, and once built allows each partner to give partial information, reduces transaction complexity, and minimizes the cost of interactions.[61] Trust builds positive expectations, intimate communication, and relationship support.[62] Safety, openness, and vulnerability are beneficial for relationships.[63]

Distrust is a different concept that shows in a negative perspective that expects disloyalty.[64] It also depletes energy because one or both people must keep track of behaviors, comments, and activities. A lack of trust causes disengagement, disinterest, inattention, avoidance, higher self-protection, and lower passion.[65] Uncertainty about one's spouse creates hypervigilance and causes one to interpret all words and actions through negative lenses.[66] It's as if you expect your lover to deceive you.

So, what do I tell my client whose husband

cheated on her? "Ditch him," I want to shout, but I don't. As a therapist, my job is not to tell people what to do, but to hold a mirror in front, so to speak, so they see how to make their own decision. In my office, tissues fill up the wastebasket, and I sit quietly. She asks, "What should I do?" "What do you want?" "I love him. I want him," she replies. "I don't want to start over. We have children." My response, "Bring him in. Let's find out what's causing this and how we can fix your marriage."

How does one repair a loss of trust? Discussion about the real or perceived injustice is necessary, and a re-orientation of the relationship. A new contract establishes the expectations, rules, and procedure for meeting needs should occur.[67]

Fidelity between people is about what you say or don't say, and what you do or don't do. It requires impeccability in words and deeds. Building trust in the beginning is much easier.

There are ways you can do this: don't make promises you're unlikely to keep, even small ones. Follow through on things. Be forthcoming with your thoughts and feelings. Refrain from hiding details from your spouse. Take risks together and open yourself. It may hurt but building relationships requires sacrificial gifts.[68] Most of all, be candid with yourself. If you are truthful to you, it is easier to be sincere with your partner.

## SPIRITUAL REFLECTION

*The Lord said to me, "Go, show your love to your wife again, though she is loved by another man and is an adulteress. Love her as the Lord loves the Israelites, though they turn to other gods and love the sacred raisin cakes.*

Hosea 3:1

If you're unfamiliar with Hosea's story, this verse is shocking. God asks Hosea to marry a promiscuous woman and have children with her. In obedience, Hosea does so, and thereby, provides a living example of Israel's unfaithfulness to God. It's one of the saddest books of scripture. It speaks to how a lack of trust de-stabilizes relationships.

What does it mean to place trust in someone? It's really a spiritual endeavor. There is absolutely no reason to trust anyone, but we do it all the time. A group became outrageous when I said, "I expect my friends or spouse will betray me at some point." They thought it was a dismal view. I thought I was being realistic.

We are humans and we are selfish at times. Even amid betrayal, even simple ones, I trust my spouse because he returns, he seeks my forgiveness, and he finds new ways to demonstrate his love. And I am the same. There are minutes when I don't honor my love and those are times when I abuse his trust in me. But, just as quickly, I seek his forgiveness so that trust is restored. Out of his love for me, and our love for one another, we restore our trust. Then we are diligent in our faithfulness to one another.

# Essential Oil: Jasmine

Distrust erodes relationships. To help in healing and rebuilding, Jasmine will help build strength as you seek support in new ways. Jasmine interacts with your emotional self by penetrating and lowering your fears while restoring a sense of trust.[69] It helps you rise above pessimism, allowing you to address problems in your relationship by creating trust.[70]

Jasmine also helps in restoring the initial infatuation, that heart flutter you first felt when meeting the love of your life when trust was natural.[71] Did you know it takes over 10 pounds of jasmine flowers to produce one 5 ml. bottle?[72] But every drop is worth it when it restores trust. You can combine it with a carrier oil to make perfume or apply to cotton balls to place in air vents around your home.[73]

## Take Action

1. Ask your partner to do a small task for you. Be sure it's something that is possible.

2. Stare into one another's eyes for 30 seconds.

3. Take turns with a blindfold leading one another someplace.

4. Play a game such as "2 Truths and a Lie." In this game each of you share 2 truths and one lie about things your partner does not about you. See if you guess which is the lie.

5. Practice effective apologies by apologizing, express remorse, and make amends.[74]

# REFLECT

How would you rate the level of trust in your relationship? In what ways has your partner demonstrated trustworthiness?

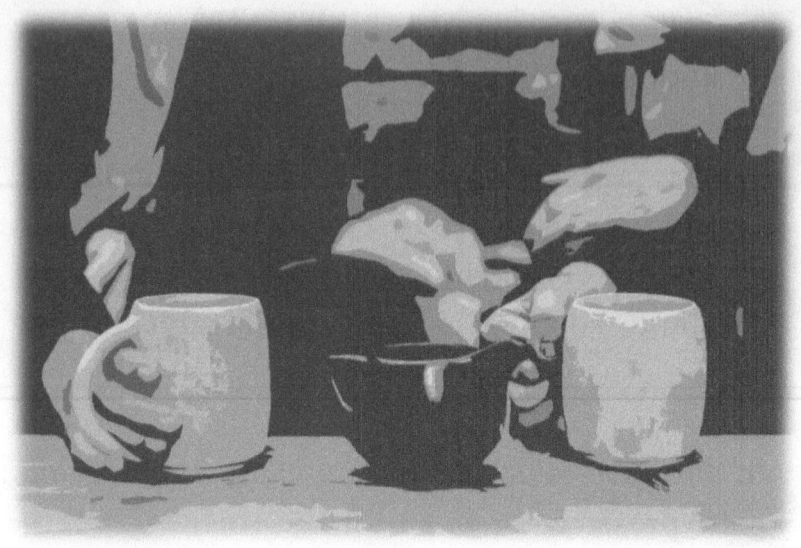

## Chapter 6
# INTIMACY

*True love is not a hide and seek game:
in true love, both lovers seek each other.*

Michael Bassey Johnson

What does it mean to be intimate with someone? Is intimacy physical? Many people fall into believing intimacy is about the act of sex. If that's the case, then we miss out on the richer context of relationships. One cannot be intimate without knowing and liking one's self, trusting and caring for one's partner, being honest, and communicating. Bockarova says intimacy requires deep knowledge of one's lover, interdependence, care, trust, responsiveness, mutuality, and commitment.[75] Being intimate requires emotional and physical affection. It's about closeness and sexuality.[76]

Wouldn't it be easier to take a pill and have instant closeness? While there are medications that help with sexual dysfunction, there are none that help you feel close to your spouse. Satisfaction arises out of positive perceptions of emotions and sex, while communication improves these.[77] In a loving relationship, sex increases intimacy and intimacy enhances sex.[78] Don't let anyone convince you that using a pill, potion, or oil will cause your sexual life to blossom. It's more complicated than that. Intimacy involves one's mind, relationship issues, emotions, and physical characteristics.[79] Yet, higher sexual satisfaction correlates with good communication, and changes over the lifetime of the relationship.[80]

Where do intimacy problems come from? Issues arise from childhood, abusive relationships, self-esteem, power inequities, and expectations. Physical problems occur with medication side effects, obesity, heart conditions, or other medical problems. Mental health is a factor as depression or anxiety decrease satisfaction. It is always best to seek a medical evaluation to rule out physical or psychological factors that play a role.

What do you expect your intimacy to be like? Most likely, closeness is different from what your lover expects. That discrepancy can create conflict. In distressed couples, fights around sexual intimacy are challenging.[81] They may be a result of low self-esteem, shame, or a sense of inadequacy.[82] Some people are perfectionists. They view sexuality as an achievement, or want to control sex, or have moralistic values around it.[83]

So, how do you develop more intimacy? A magic potion won't help. Closeness, desire, and satisfaction take creativity, commitment, and time. You must run towards your spouse, not away from him or her. Instead of turning away, you need to turn in, press through, and find the common ground.

Sexual intimacy builds throughout the day as you are playful with one another, as you pay attention to each other, and as you interact positively.[84] Recapture your dating behaviors. Flirt again and allow tension to build. Focus on affectionate touch—hold hands more often. Make time for one another. Be emotionally vulnerable during sex while maintaining a sense of curiosity. Vary the type of sex you have with your loved one. Ask for what you need, instead of telling what you don't want.[85]

Intimacy is being comfortable with your partner and meeting his or her basic needs with honesty and respect. Commit to bringing your lover joy and fun each day. Develop your private language and inside jokes. Use personal signals to play with one another.[86] Talk often and openly with your spouse. And, don't forget to cuddle.[87]

## SPIRITUAL REFLECTION

*Place me like a seal over your heart, like a seal on your arm; for love is as strong as death, its jealousy unyielding as the grave. It burns like blazing fire, like a mighty flame. Many waters cannot quench love; rivers cannot sweep it away. If one were to give all the wealth of one's house for love, it would be utterly scorned.*

Song of Songs 8:6-7

We are wonderful creations. Our physical desire comes from a brain that connects our heart, soul, and emotions. We are not biological primates who use sexuality only for propagation. It is the combination of all of these that give us intimacy. Animals do not share that same level of closeness that we do. Yet, we find so many ways to disrupt it.

Our natural tendencies are self-serving. We can call it survival but the true way we conquer life is through our connections with each other. We cannot do this alone. It is the echo of Genesis 2 that repeats in the Song of Songs. This longing is unquenchable and only finds its completion as we rediscover one another and the Creator. Allow yourself to awaken within, freeing your senses and your wishes. Become like the lovers in Song of Songs. Draw near to one another.

## ESSENTIAL OIL: NEROLI

Neroli has a sweet scent. This oil comes from the orange blossom and is common in France, Italy, and Morroco.[88] First distilled in the 16th century, neroli is named after the Italian princess of Nerola, Anna Maria de la Tremoille.[89] This essential oil enhances creativity and releases energy.[90] It helps you connect your soul and spirit, increasing your sense of satisfaction.[91] Mojay says neroli is both sensual and spiritual.[92]

Neroli makes sense when you understand what intimacy entails and the importance of connecting body, mind, and spirit. Use it in your bath or diffuser to relax and calm you. Allow the connection between your inner self help you in your joining with your loved one.

## TAKE ACTION

Here are some fun activities to increase intimacy.

1. Find a sex questionnaire in a magazine and complete it together.

2. Explore different ways of kissing.

3. Practice breathing together. Lean your head against your partner's head and breathe in and out, matching breaths.

4. Share something with your spouse that he or she doesn't know about you.

## REFLECT

When do you feel the most intimate? What acts increase your intimacy? What actions during the day create more excitement for you about your partner?

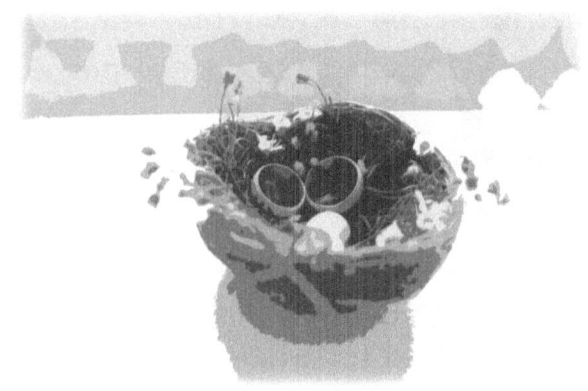

# Chapter 7
# COMMITMENT

*If we commit ourselves to one person for life, this is not, as many people think, a rejection of freedom; rather, it demands the courage to move into all the risks of freedom, and the risk of love which is permanent; into that love which is not possession but participation.*

Madeleine L'Engle

What does commitment mean? Is it insistence on one partner for life? Or for as long as one feels a sense of love? Perhaps commitment says if you treat me right, then I will stay with you. Are vows meaningful? Think about the last wedding you attended, and the words exchanged between the lovers.

Sometimes in public ceremonies, couples write their own pledges. I remember sitting with my fiancé and discussing the oath. Then we spoke with the minister. While we wanted to use a traditional pledge, there were parts of it we wanted to exclude, like "obey." That word seemed more like a command between a parent and child, not two loving adults. For sure we included "for better or worse, in sickness and health, until death do us part." We wanted to believe that this is possible. However, it's harder to live out than to speak.

For some people, commitment is directly related to an investment model. As long as I'm satisfied and receive a positive return, then I'm willing to stay with my partner.[93] For other couples, this promise is an intention to persist despite difficulties, or to make it for the long-haul, or at least as long as they experience a strong psychological attachment.[94] Whatever the two believe, commitment is a dynamic process that continually changes throughout the course of a lifetime. It means re-constructing the relationship occasionally.[95]

In studies of commitment, there are three themes that emerge: desire, duty, and obligation.[96] The desire to remain with a person is personal and comes from a positive attitude about one's relationship. Whereas duty arises out of a moral responsibility or religious belief that involves self-constraint.[97] Obligation occurs when one realizes the investment, and one's initial payment cannot be returned. Or, one stays because of fear of social reactions, difficulties in leaving, or because someone better is not available.[98]

Whatever the reason, partners soon realize that continuing means that each must accommodate the needs of the other and offer sacrifices.[99] How spouses view this vow matters. Those who have good memories last. It also means accepting one's partner, warts and all. I tell clients choosing a lover is choosing a set of problems. You cannot escape trials because there is no perfect person. It's a myth to think otherwise.

So, how can people maintain their commitment? Part of it is acceptance. You will have a conflict. That's natural and can strengthen the relationship. You need ways to connect daily that involve little rituals like the goodbye kiss, a little wave, or the "hello, are you home?"[100] Remaining present requires perseverance, responsibility, and devotion.[101]

It means leaving is not an option. Commitment is good for relationships. When it is strong, satisfaction increases and partners become more invested.[102] When I rule out separation or divorce, I must make this relationship work because I depend on you and you need me.[103]

How can you fortify your resolve? Accommodating a partner's needs or sacrificing for the good of the relationship are vital. Forgiveness and shifting from a "what's good for me" orientation to "what's best for us" helps. It means being thankful and comparing the good things you have as compared to those people who don't have those. And, it includes an awareness that someone different isn't better.[104] Communicating commitment means reassuring my partner by stating my feelings, encouraging them, paying attention to their needs and interests. It happens in the ways that I do tangible things like giving gifts, love notes, or doing small acts of kindness. Celebrations of milestones and keeping promises show my loved one they matter to me.[105]

We live in a world of instant gratification with ready-made delicious meals and free access to almost any gratuitous privilege. While those are wonderful, they also lure us into thinking relationships must operate the same way. The way to maintain commitment means that we understand the permanency of "us," and we don't give up amid the turbulence that arises when facing life's storms. Instead, we drop anchor and hold onto one another, viewing each other as fellow sailors on a stormy sea that are seeking to survive. And, when the calm arrives, we congratulate ourselves because we made it through together. What a wonderful way to live!

# Spiritual Reflection

*Two are better than one, because they have a good return for their labor: if either of them falls down, one can help the other up . . . if two lied down together, they will keep warm . . . Though one may be overpowered, two can defend themselves. A cord of three strands is not quickly broken.*

Ecclesiastes 4:9, 10a, 11a, 12

This is such a focused example of what commitment looks like. However, notice how the three-fold cord is strongest. Guess who needs to be the strongest and final part of the strand? Without a spiritual connection to the Holy One, the relationship has less strength. Partners must be woven together along with a spiritual commitment to God.

As I reflect on 40 years of marriage, I cannot imagine how it is possible for lovers to stay together without God. Sometimes I wasn't sure I would make it through the difficult times, but I would pray, "Lord, help me understand him. Let me see things through his eyes. Give me patience and love." I'm sure he did the same with me. That binding reminds us that we must remain strong together. So often in counseling, I remind couples. You are not enemies. The foe is something outside of you: worries, finances, circumstances, other people, etc. The key is to remember you are allies and you win by joining in a fight of that which tries to separate you.

At one point, my mom posted a sticker on her car that said, "The family that prays together stays together." I recall how cheesy that seemed. My friends laughed at the sign. How little I realized the significance of that silly statement. Sometimes my husband told me, "I'm praying for you." It made my heart melt that he included me in his prayers. It reminded me we are in this together with the One who loves us dearly. Looking back, I can see all the times that our commitment kept us steady, guiding us through our trials. And, it will continue to do so.

## ESSENTIAL OIL: VETIVER

Commitment serves as a base of any relationship. When life brings disappointments, hurts, or disruptions, and we doubt our choices, our partner, or our relationship, we need something to reinforce the foundation. It's difficult to do so when feeling uneasy with one's partner.

Vetiver is an essential oil which connects us to the solid earth. It reminds us of the ground beneath us.[106] Vetiver comes from a grass native to India and helps prevent soil erosion around the world,[107] bringing us in touch with that which grounds us and frees us to receiving what others offer. It helps clear our confusion while reinforcing boundaries.[108] Worwood says it settles the swirl of questions and brings a sense of calm amid instability.[109] Use in baths, or in a diffuser, or try rubbing some on the bottom of your feet to help ground you.

# Take Action

Try some of the following activities to strengthen the foundation of your relationship and your commitment to one another.

1. Do more things together: read a book, travel,

or take a class.

2. Volunteer together at a homeless shelter or other non-profit organization.

3. Write a mission statement for the next year or five years. What do you want to accomplish together?

4. Take up a new sport together like hiking. Explore new areas in your location.

# REFLECT

What does commitment mean to you? In what ways do you show loyalty to your partner? What is one thing you can do to affirm your pledge to your loved one this week?

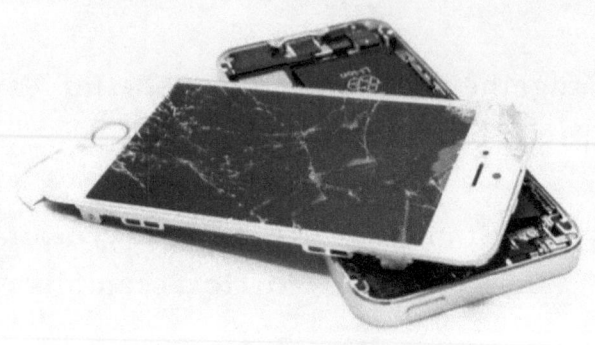

Chapter 8

# COMMUNICATION

*Listen with curiosity. Speak with honesty. Act with integrity. The greatest problem with communication is we don't listen to understand. We listen to reply. When we listen with curiosity, we don't listen with the intent to reply. We listen for what's behind the words.*

Roy T. Bennett

Tempting as it is to leave this chapter to the quote above without further remarks, there are some ideas that require further comments. Most of us assume we can talk. Some realize we get stuck around sensitive issues. Few understand how to navigate through those difficult conversations.

Google "communication in marriages," and you will get over 58,000,000 results. There's no shortage of information. Yet, why do you struggle with your loved one? Every couple in therapy gets at least one session dedicated to conflict resolution. Yet most duos will find marriage counseling ineffective and drop out prematurely.[110]

When things are going well, talking isn't a problem unless you or your partner have lost your concern for one another. Maintaining positivity in a relationship is critical. It's easy to take your spouse for granted. When you do so, you stop thinking of things about them you admire. Appreciation decreases, and you notice their irritating habits. Once you key in on those, it's hard to refocus and you distance yourself. Before you know it, you're either "picking" at your partner's faults or you've "written the person off." A negative attitude sets in along with disillusionment. It doesn't have to be that way. But it requires a deliberate focus on reminding yourself about your loved one's best features.[111]

In going through marital therapy at one point, I thought my husband and I were on the edge of divorce. The counselor reassured me we were not even close. She helped me refocus on what I loved about him when she pointed out that we had so much in common. That redirection helped save my marriage.

Even having a positive regard for your lover doesn't mean that every day is wonderful. There will be times of stress and disagreement. In fact, John Gottman and his team find that 69% of conflict persists in relationships.[112] That leaves couples either at an impasse or forced to re-learn how to discuss things.[113] It's imperative you recognize what creates a meaningful conversation or you'll end up where you started, back in gridlock. In distressed couples, poor communication indicates lower marital happiness.[114] Roy Bennett has the right idea.[115]

The recipe for a successful discussion must include curiosity, honesty, integrity, selflessness, and earnest listening.

Let's explore why most counseling doesn't work. When couples see a therapist, they spend time explaining when, how, and why they disagree. During this conversation, the lovers show how they get stuck in conversation without realizing they're doing so. If the therapist does not interrupt, and allows them to continue, they waste the hour. Sometimes the spouses insist on continuing to argue in the session, not allowing intervention. One couple did this, despite my repeated efforts to redirect them. When they ran out of steam near the end of our time, I said, "You just paid me $135 to listen to you fight. Was it worth it?" Therapy in this manner will be meaningless because it reinforces a negative pattern.

So, what does good communication involve? First, it requires a desire to understand one's lover. Even amid strife, the goal needs to be seeing the other person's perspective. It doesn't mean agreement. If I love someone, I will listen to get a sense of his or her core concern. That means I move from thinking of how I'll respond, defending my position, or trying to express my opinion, and instead concentrate on my spouse. What is his most basic need? Is it reassurance, connection, or support? I can offer those without agreeing with his view.

Healthy discourse occurs when I refrain from using a negative filter. If he says, "I like your hair better today," I don't determine whether that's a positive or negative statement. Instead, I view it as a neutral observation. Too often I interpret the other person's words or actions as offensive and then feel slighted. If I view them as neither negative nor positive, but somewhere in between, it helps me maintain a sense of balance. Gottman calls this positive sentiment override.[116]

So, where do problems come from? If most issues will be perpetual, how can couples succeed? Communication is about behaviors, intentions, tone, body language, and words. Breakdowns occur when we don't show care or when we're only interested in having our way. When we approach our spouses with a harsh, demeaning, or demanding tone, we lose their attention.

Words matter. When accusatory, our partners become defensive. Communication suffers when we're insincere, impatient, nagging, over-reactive, or unkind.[117] Our busy-ness distances us and we forget to attend to our lover's needs.

So, what helps? Being open and receiving influence from our spouse will improve the relationship. Communication gets better when we respect and listen for understanding. When we clarify information before reacting, we prevent misunderstanding.[118] It means changing the current pattern to something different.

## Spiritual Reflection

*A gentle answer turns away wrath, but a harsh word stirs up anger.*

Proverbs 15:1

*The heart of the righteous weighs its answers, but the mouth of the wicked gushes evil.*

Proverbs 15:28

How often have you said something and wished to take it back? Unfortunately, it's out in the open and doing its damage. Many snags in marriages are avoided when one pauses before responding. My son observed this many times as my husband hesitated in answering a question I posed or to my complaint about something. He asked about the silence, and my husband explained sometimes there is no correct answer. "When that happens, you must think before you say anything. Sometimes it's a no-win situation." How wise.

My advice to people is thinking before they speak. I need to practice this more because I know it works better. I'm reminded of Jesus' hesitation to reply to accusations. When he did respond, he didn't defend himself. He redirected the conversation back to the speaker, asking questions that made them reflect. Isn't that what we need when our partner is upset? The more we are still and calm, the better we become at listening and meeting one another's needs. When that happens, the other person settles down and we come to a mutual agreement about how we can proceed.

# ESSENTIAL OIL: CLARY SAGE

To calm the mind and decrease emotional tension, clary sage is a wonderful choice.[119] It creates a slight euphoria, lifting one's spirit and energy to help in difficult times.[120] Clary sage helps bring clarity about issues and enhances our natural intuition.[121] This oil can be used in a compress, as an ointment when combined with a carrier, or inhaled. Try some before your next difficult conversation.

# TAKE ACTION

Try these to enhance your communication.

1. Don't assume. Instead, approach your partner with a sense of curiosity. Say, "Tell me what's going on."

2. When you offer feedback, point out things your spouse is doing right. Remember,

positive reinforcement works better.

3. Choose your timing correctly. Ask yourself, "Is this a good time to bring this up, or should I wait?"[122]

4. When you have a disagreement, focus on the current issue. Don't bring up past situations.

# REFLECT

What prevents you from being honest with your partner? How can you show your spouse that you want to understand his/her perspective?

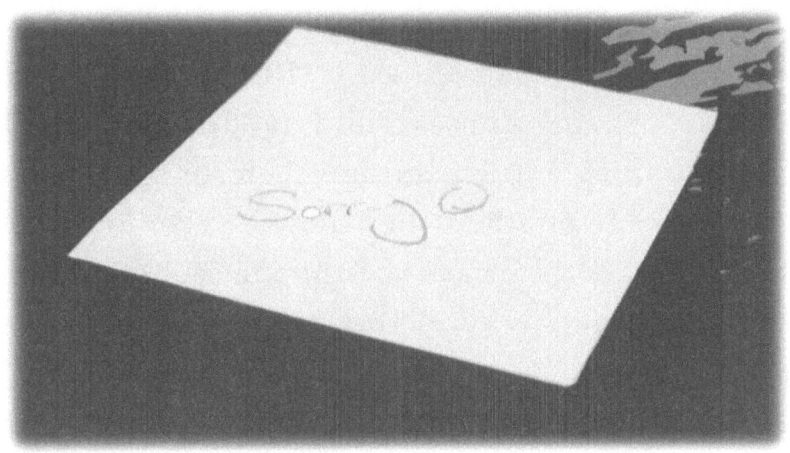

## Chapter 9

*Forgiveness is an act of the will, and the will can function regardless of the temperature of the heart.*

Corrie Ten Boom

The two most important words in a relationship are "I'm sorry." Yet saying these aloud is difficult. As I coach couples and encourage them to speak this phrase to one another, they almost seem to choke on them as if they have a fishbone stuck in their parched throat. Why is this so hard? Marriages fare better when partners acknowledge responsibility for mistakes, harsh words, or unloving acts. Marital happiness increases when couples practice forgiveness.[123]

There are many studies of marital forgiveness; all finding the practice is a powerful protective factor.[124] When lovers are forgiving, they have more positive assumptions and better communication.[125] Miller and Worthington found men are more forgiving and wives perceive their husbands as more forgiving. Forgiveness creates trust.[126]

But, wait a minute, you say. If it's that easy, then why are things so wrong in my relationship? Is it enough to say, "I'm sorry"? You already know that answer, don't you? It's not. Words are meaningless unless accountability and action accompany them. When one spouse injures another and then offers an apology, it is a step in the right direction. But several more steps must follow.

Many partners will say, "I didn't hurt her" or "I didn't mean to offend him". The first statement neglects responsibility and the latter comment considers intention an excuse. Neither is sufficient, nor are they helpful in making amends. Whether we injure someone is not for us to decide. We are working with our partner's perception. If we love and respect them, we will honor their view of things. If my spouse says, "You hurt me," then it's true. He's describing his experience and needs me to acknowledge his wound. If I say, "Well, I didn't mean to hurt you," it's an effort to repair but does not take away his pain. Think of it this way. If I reach out and slap you, it will hurt. When you say, "Ouch! That hurt. Why did you do that?" and I respond, "Oh, I'm sorry. I didn't intend to hit you," it doesn't make things right. You're still sore. I must take it further and offer a sincere apology that tells you I see you hurting, I am guilty of doing that to you, I deeply regret my action, and I promise to change. I do not want to hurt you again.

That's the first part of the reconciliatory process. The second half belongs to you. The choice becomes yours. Either you will or won't exonerate me. Here is where I remind my clients that forgiveness is a thought and an action. It is not a feeling. You must state, "I forgive you," and then act as if you have done so. It's hard, I know. You may say, "But I don't *feel* better. I still hurt." Yes, I understand. You may have to practice forgiveness every day. When you awake, say, "I forgive him or her. I will treat him or her as if I have forgiven him or her." Forgiveness is not instantaneous. It unfolds over time.

A word of caution is necessary. If you offer forgiveness too quickly after an incident, it can backfire. It lets your lover "off the hook" and prevents him or her from making changes. If there are no consequences, then he or she will probably repeat the same behavior.[127] This can be dangerous in relationships with physical and emotional aggression. A spouse who is too quick to forgive will have a partner who continues to act in unloving ways.[128] While you ought to forgive, allow some time, perhaps 24 hours, before you offer forgiveness. Doing so provides you and your loved one a "cooling off" period allowing contemplation. The conversation that follows is more fruitful.

So, how does one practice forgiveness in a relationship? What critical elements facilitate the process? According to Fife and colleagues, reconciliation includes empathy, humility, commitment, and hope.[129] Everett Worthington developed a model called REACH, an acronym for recall, empathize, altruism, committing, and holding on. One remembers the hurt objectively (recall) and attempts to understand the viewpoint of the one who hurt them (empathize). Offering altruism occurs when you remember times when you hurt someone and were forgiven, thereby offering forgiveness to the person who is hurting you. Committing means publicly forgiving your offender and holding on reminds you to remember the pain, but also your choice to forgive.[130] It isn't easy, but you can do it.

# Spiritual Reflection

*Therefore, as God's chosen people, holy and dearly loved, clothe yourselves with compassion, kindness, humility, gentleness and patience. Bear with each other and forgive one another if any of you has a grievance against someone. Forgive as the Lord forgave you. And over all of these virtues put on love, which binds them all together in perfect unity.*

Colossians 3:12—14

Something seems so simple but difficult to practice. Why bother with forgiveness? The benefits of forgiveness are worth the effort. It will strengthen your love, it will set you free, and it teaches us how to offer forgiveness to others.[131] The practice of forgiveness keeps us mentally and physically healthy.[132] Think of how many times we hurt others and the ways they offer mercy to us. It's a blessing to receive compassion despite our mistakes and failures.

How do you begin? Uglow[133] makes the following recommendations:

1. Decide to forgive. You have a choice. You

don't have to offer forgiveness. And forgiveness doesn't mean that you will forget the event. When wounded, it seems like you lose control. In realizing you have a choice, power returns to you.

2. One thing at a time. Start with the small things and stay current. If your lover does something today, for example, forget to run an errand for you, forgive that mistake. Don't let the little things build until they become overwhelming.

3. Accept the pain. Ouch. I know that hurt. But, when you face the sting, you increase your strength.

4. Look for the positive lesson. I don't mean to sound trite here, but I want you to realize that this can bring growth to you.

5. Practice empathy. This relates to the REACH model. Put yourself in your spouse's shoes. Try to understand his reasoning.

6. Be compassionate. That's the essence of

what the apostle Paul is saying in this passage. You and your partner are the body of Christ. Forgive him or her just as Christ forgave you when you least deserved it.

## Essential Oil: Helichrysum

Unforgiveness is unhealthy in many ways. It prevents us from reaching out to those most helpful in our time of hurt. It also causes immobilization, leaving us unable to process our wounds, or deal with those who hurt us. For this, helichrysum (Everlasting) is effective in helping restore the balance.

Helichrysum is from the Everlasting shrub which grows to 22 inches in height. It is found in the Mediterranean basin and is also known as the "Italian straw flower."[134] Helichrysum is useful for people who experience emotional blocking.[135] The oil can untie the tightest knots within the self, restoring one's ability to think clearly.[136]

# TAKE ACTION

Here are some ways to practice forgiveness:

1. Write an apology letter. That gives you time to form your words carefully. In the letter, acknowledge your role, how it wounded your partner, your intention, regret, and promise for the future.

2. Imagine a 3rd party who is objective but desires the best for your relationship. This person doesn't side with either of you. What would this person say to you?
3. Talk with your spouse about what forgiveness means to you. Ask what it means to them. Try to see each other's point of view.

# REFLECT

What do you think forgiveness entails? Have you been forgiven by someone? What did they do or say? What thoughts and feelings arise when you focus on that forgiveness? How can you use that with your loved one.

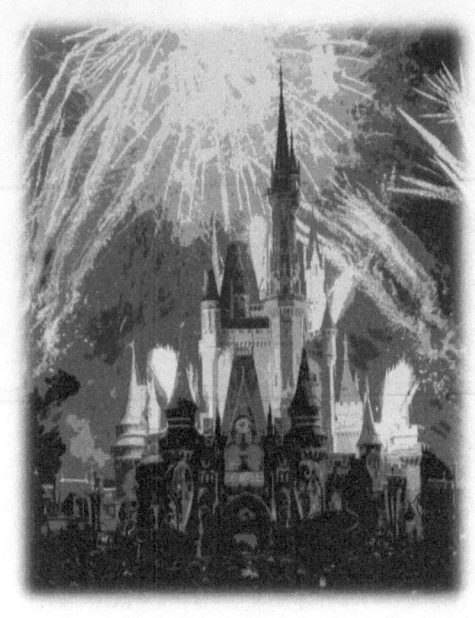

## Chapter 10
# HAPPILY, AFTER ALL

*And they lived happily (aside from a few normal disagreements, misunderstandings, pouts, silent treatments, and unexpected calamities) ever after.*

Jean Farris

The handsome prince kisses the sleeping beauty and they live. Isn't that the best part? They live together. And in living, they find love, and joy, and strife, and growth. That's the beauty of this wonderful thing called "relationship," "marriage," and "love." It's alive and ever changing. Who wants the same story every day?

Some struggle with this idea that marriage or romance doesn't last forever. It's important to realize that we have problems. From 1990 to 2004, half of all U.S. marriages ended in divorce.[137] In recent years, the divorce rate is decreasing in adults younger than 39, primarily because they are delaying marriage until certain it will last. However, it is still twice the rate of those who are over 40 years of age. The sadder news is that dissolution of marriages is rising sharply among adults over 50 due to decreasing marital satisfaction.[138] Overall, the U.S. divorce rate remains about 50%.[139] So, we still have a problem.

Why does marriage fail? Why are the first five years so important? One reason relates back to the myth love relationships will fulfill all our needs.[140] But, it doesn't. There's no fairy tale, no magic potion, no godmother with a twinkling wand to rescue the lovers from the burning castle. When the prince and princess fight, it's a duel to see who wins, and someone always gets hurt. They forget they live in the same kingdom and must become fierce allies lest an outside enemy steal their treasures.

Another reason for divorce relates to family dynamics. When you join with another human being, you become part of a larger system, a family, and that is unavoidable. Even if you and your partner vow to cut yourselves off from your families, their voices, principles, and values still circle in your heads. They tell you who should take out the trash, who pays the bills, how you should treat a person, and how the partner should treat you. You cannot escape that.

A third reason is a different plan for life.[141] When couples come for counseling, I ask if they're on the same train. They look at me as if I have two heads. I say, "If you, Bill, are on a train to Chicago, and Nancy is on a train to San Francisco, then we've got trouble." I explain the importance of having similar goals, values, traditions, and spiritual beliefs. Marriage is the train and it cannot jump tracks just to suit one's impulsive desires or change in contract.

Recently a couple appeared before me. They were having an ongoing argument, which isn't unusual, but as we explored further, the disagreement was a change in the relationship contract. Early on, he said he would never ask his partner to do X but now he asked her to do X. In the beginning, she told him she would never do X. As she was shaking with fear and anger, she said, "I meant what I said back then. But now I feel like if I don't give in, you'll call it quits." I stopped them and pointed out he was trying to re-negotiate a business contract, but it appeared more like a hostile takeover. He understood the business analogy. I asked if that's how he would handle a work contract. He said, "Of course not. I'd lose the business." I just smiled and then he said, "Ooh, I see." Yes, good. It's important to be on the same train going to the same destination.

A fourth reason relationships fail is because of a pattern of disconnection.[142] This happens gradually. People get busy and forget to stay on top of their marriage. I say to couples, "There is no auto-pilot in marriage. If you're not working on it, you're losing the relationship." So many people come into the counseling office and tell me work is too pressing, the kids are the priority, financial stability is vital, and a lot of other rationalizations for ignoring their connection. No, *stop right now*. Your marriage is the most important thing. What will you have once you retire? Who stays with you after the kids leave? The investment is costly but will pay substantial dividends if you continue to invest in your commitment.

These factors play a role. Above all of these, Dr. John Gottman says there is one thing that predicts an untimely and unwelcome demise to love. Dr. Gottman has a 90% accuracy record in predicting divorce and can do so in a matter of minutes by observing the communication pattern. He calls this negative set of interactions "The Four Horsemen of the Apocalypse."[143] These include criticism of one's partner, contempt or a strong sense of dislike and mocking, defensiveness, and stonewalling.[144] When couples appear for counseling, I look for that unrelenting pattern and interrupt it. I explain I will do this, and sometimes be controlling with how and when partners talk with one another. My goal is to intervene at the moment and show the individuals a different way to interact. Couples are amazed at how this alters their relationship. But I need them in my office before I can help them.

The last reason relationships fail is because couples wait five to six years after spotting a problem before they seek help. When they arrive, they want the problem solved in 3–4 sessions. That's a trap for everyone. Even then, only 37% of couples will seek help before divorcing, and when they do, few receive evidence-based treatments, leading to a marital counseling failure.[145] That's why this book exists. It's not a substitute for therapy, but it provides some tips for enhancing your relationship.

When talking with others about love, I like to use Gottman's analogy of a house.[146] He says that load-bearing walls must be trust and commitment, while the foundation is marital friendship. The first level up is fondness and admiration while the second floor is turning towards one another instead of away. The next level is maintaining a positive perspective and moving up to the sixth floor where conflict management occurs. My favorite level, though, is the top, which I call the penthouse. That level is where dreams come true and together couples create meaningful lives.[147] If, and that's a very big if, fairy tales really do come true, they happen at this stage. But there are a lot of steps to climb in-between the floors of the house. But, maybe it's possible.

With hope, and a whole lot of effort, I will see you waving from the penthouse. In the meantime, I want to encourage you to continue to seek ways to love one another. Don't give up. Relationships go through cycles. Some years may not be as good as other years. Spend time caring for one another, practicing patience, self-sacrifice, and praying a lot. If you follow these suggestions, you will be *happily* married, *after all.*

## Resources Cited

Ackerman, C. E. (2019). 21 couples therapy worksheets, techniques, & activities.

Alderson, M. (2019). The end is the beginning.

Algoe, S. B., Kurtz, L. E., & Grewen, K. (2017, Aug.). Oxytocin and social bonds: The role of oxytocin in perceptions of romantic partners' bonding behavior. *Psychological Science, 28*(12).

Arangua, M. (2018, Dec 20). How to tell if you have an intimate relationship.

Barry, R. A., Lawrence, E., & Langer, A. (2008). Conceptualization and assessment of disengagement in romantic relationships. *Personal Relationships, 15*, 297-315.

Battaglia, S. (2003). *Complete guide to aromatherapy*. Brisbane, Australia: Perfect Potion.

Battaglia, S. (2019, Jan 2). Ylang ylang monograph. *Salvatore Battaglia.*
Battaglia, S. (2018, May 9). Neroli. *Salvatore*

*Battaglia.*

Bellows, A. (2018, Oct 8). Good communication in marriage starts with respect. *PsychCentral*

Bloom, L., & Bloom, C. (2016, Apr 29). The art of friendship in marriage. *Psychology Today.*

Bockarova, M. (2018, Feb 14). The 7 elements that define an intimate relationship. *Psychology Today.*

Bonior, A. (2018, Dec 12). 7 ways to build trust in a relationship. *Psychology Today.*

Bronzite, D. (2019). The hero's journey – mythic structure of Joseph Campbell's monomyth.

Campbell, L., Boldry, J. G., Simpson, J. A., & Rubin, H. (2010). Trust, variability in relationship evaluations, and relationship processes. *Journal of Personality & Social Psychology, 99*(1), 14-31.

Cohen, E. D. (2019). Perfect in bed: Demanding sexual perfection can destroy your sex life. *Psychology Today, 52*(5), 34-36.

Cohen, M. (2016, Dec 14). The importance of physical affection for relationship satisfaction. *Luvze.*

Dashnaw, D. (2018, May 18). 13 best ways to show respect in marriage. *Couples Therapy Inc.*

Davis, P. (1991). *Subtle aromatherapy.* Saffron Walden, England: The C. W. Daniel Company.

Elmore, L. (2019). 10 ways to use cinnamon bark.

Emery, L. R. (2017, May 22). 15 little ways to improve communication in your relationship. *Bustle.*

Feuerman, M. (2017, Apr 6). The danger of sliding instead of deciding to get married. *The Gottman Institute.*

Fischer-Rizzi, S. (1991). *Complete aromatherapy handbook: Essential oil for radiant health.* New York, NY: Sterling Publishing Co.

Floyd, K., Hess, J. A., Miczo, L. A., Halone, K. K., Mikkelson, A. C., & Tusing, K. J. (2005). Human affection exchange: VIII: Further evidence of the benefits of expressed affection. *Communication Quarterly, 53*, 285-303.

Floyd, K., Boren, J. P., Hannaway, A. F., Hesse, C., McEwan, B., & Veksler, A. E. (2009). Kissing in marital and cohabiting relationships: Effects on blood lipids, stress, and relationship satisfaction. *Western Journal of Communication, 73*(2), 113-133.

Frank, E., & Brandsttäter, V. (2002). Approach versus avoidance: Different types of commitment in intimate relationships. *Journal of Personality and Social Psychology, 82*(2), 208-221.

Gaspard, T. (2016, Dec. 7). 10 ways to rekindle the passion in your marriage. *The Gottman Institute.*

Gottman, J. M. (2011). *The science of trust: Emotional attunement for couples.* New York, NY: W.W. Norton & Company.

Gottman, J. (2019). Marriage and couples. *The*

*Gottman Institute.*

Gottman, J. M., & Gottman, J. (2019, Jan 30). The eight conversations that matter most in relationships. *The Gottman Institute.*

Gottman, J. M., & Silver, N. (2000). *The seven principles for making marriage work: A practical guide from the country's foremost relationship expert.* New York, NY: Three Rivers Press.

Guinness World Book of Records. (2015, Feb 12). Valentine's Day: Ten of the most romantic world records.

Guilbault, V., & Philippe, F. L. (2017). Commitment in romantic relationships as a function of partners' encoding of important couple-related memories. *Memory, 25*(5), 595-606.

Gulledge, A. K., Gulledge, M.H., & Stahmann, R. F. (2003). Romantic physical affection types and relationship satisfaction. *American Journal of Family Therapy, 31*(4), 233-242.

Helm, B. (2017, Fall). Friendship. In *The Stanford encyclopedia of philosophy.*

Hendrick, C., Hendrick, S. S., & Zacchilli, T. L. (2011). Respect and love in romantic relationships. *Acta de Investigación Psicológica, 1*(2), 316-329.

Hendrick, S. S., & Hendrick, C. (2006). Measuring respect in close relationships. *Journal of Social and Personal Relationships, 23*(6), 881-899.

Higgins, L. (2016, Dec 19). 5 simple ways to strengthen the friendship in your marriage. *The Gottman Institute.*

Institute for Comparative Survey Research. (2018). WVS Wave 7. Vienna, Austria.

Josephs, L. (2018). Conclusion: Why people remain faithful. In *The dynamics of infidelity: Applying relationship science to psychotherapy practice* (p. 221-229). Washington, DC: American Psychological Association.

Kessler, M. (2015). The importance of commitment in intimate relationships and how to strengthen it (dissertation). University of Zurich: Zurich, Switzerland.

Khalifian, C. E., & Barry, R. A. (2016). Trust,

attachment, and mindfulness influence intimacy and disengagement during newlyweds' discussions of relationship transgressions. *Journal of Family Psychology, 30*(5), 592-601.

Lavner, J. A., Karney, B. R., & Bradbury, T. N. (2016). Does couples' communication predict marital satisfaction, or does marital satisfaction predict communication? *Journal of Marriage and Family,* (3), 680.

Lee, B., & Little, J. (1999). *Artist of life.* North Clarendon, VT: Tuttle Publishing.

Lenbuck, J. (2018, Jul 8). How does sex differ from intimacy? *PsychCentral.*

Lewicki, R. J., & Wiethoff, C. (2000). Trust, trust development, and trust repair. In M. Deutsch & P. T. Coleman, *The handbook of conflict resolution: Theory and practice* (p. 86-107). San Francisco, CA: Jossey-Bass.

Loughran, J., & Bull, R. (1997). *Aromatherapy & subtle energy techniques.* Berkeley, CA: North Atlantic Books.

Loughran, J., & Bull, R. (2001). *Aromatherapy anointing oils*. Berkeley, CA: Frog Publishing.

McKenna, W. (2017, Jun 23). In marriage, friendship triumphs over love. *Mind&Spirit*.

Meston, C. M., & Stanton, A. M. (2019). Sexuality and intimacy. In *APA handbook of contemporary family psychology: Family therapy and training, Vol. 3*(p. 325-340). Washington, DC: American Psychological Association.

Mojay, G. (1999). *Aromatherapy for healing the spirit: Restoring emotional and mental balance with essential oils.* Rochester, VT: Healing Arts Press.

Murray, S. L., Holmes, J. G., & Collins, N. L. (2006). Optimizing assurance: The risk regulation system in relationships. *Psychological Bulletin, 132*, 641-666.

Papp, L. M., Goeke-Morey, M. C., & Cummings, E. M. (2013). Let's talk about sex: A diary investigation of couples' intimacy conflicts in the home. *Couple and Family Psychology: Research and Practice, 2*(1), 34-36.

Pauley, P. M., Hesse, C., & Mikkelson, A. C. (2014). Trait affection predicts married couples' use of relational maintenance behaviors. *Journal of Family Communication, 14*(2), 167-187.

Poivre, M., & Duez, P. (2017, Mar). Biological activity and toxicity of the Chinese herb *Melissa officinalis* Rehder & E. Wilson (Houpo) and its constituents. *Journal of Zhejiang University Science B, 18*(3), 194-214.

Saad, L. (2018, May 18). Gallup vault: Fidelity, respect rates keys to marital bliss. *Gallup.*

Schneiderman, I., Zagoory-Sharon, O., Leckman, J. F., & Feldman, R. (2012, Aug). Oxytocin during the initial stages of romantic attachment: Relations to couples' interactive reciprocity. *Psychoneuroendocrinology, 37*(8), 1277-1285.

Schoebi, D., Karney, B. R., & Bradbury, T. N. (2012). Stability and change in the first 10 years of marriage: Does commitment confer benefits beyond the effects of satisfaction? *Journal of Personality and Social Psychology, 102*(4), 729-742.

Seal, K. L., Doherty, W. J., & Harris, S. M. (2015). Confiding about problems in marriage and long-term committed relationships: A national study. *Journal of Marital and Family Therapy, 42*(3), 438-450.

Seppala, E. (2012, Feb 14). Discovering the secrets of long-term love. *Scientific American.*

Theiss, J. A., & Soloman, D. H. (2006). A relational turbulence model of communication about irritations in romantic relationships. *Communication Research, 33*(5), 391.418.

Uwom-Ajaegbu, O., Ajike, E., Fadolapo, L, & Ajaegbu, C. (2015). An empirical study on the causes and effects of communication breakdown in marriages. *Journal of Philosophy, Culture and Religion, 11,* 1-9.

Weigel, D. J., & Ballard-Reisch, D. S. (2014). Constructing commitment in intimate relationships: Mapping interdependence in the everyday expressions of commitment. *Communication Research, 41*(3), 311-332.

What % of your life is spent kissing? (2019). *HappyWorker.*

Whitbourne, S. K. (2014, Jan 28). Seven types of physical affection in relationships. *Psychology Today.*

Worwood, V. A. (1996). *The fragrant mind: Aromatherapy for personality, mind, mood, and emotion.* Novato, CA: New World Library.

Wudarczyk, O. A., Earp, B. D., Guastella, A., & Savulescu, J. (2013, Sep). Could intranasal oxytocin be used to enhance relationships? Research imperatives, clinical policy, and ethical considerations. *Current Opinion in Psychiatry, 26*(5), 474-484.

Yoo, H., Bartle-Haring, S., Day, R. D., & Gangamma, R. (2014). Couple communication, emotional and sexual intimacy, and relationship satisfaction. *Journal of Sex & Marital Therapy, 40*(4), 275-293.

Young Living Essential Oils. (2019). All about jasmine [blog].

Zeck, R. (2008). *The blossoming heart: Aromatherapy for healing and transformation.* Victoria, Australia: Aroma Tours.

# ABOUT THE AUTHORS

Kathy Hoppe is a licensed marital & family therapist, amateur artist, adjunct faculty member, minister, certified compassion fatigue specialist, and certified Aroma Freedom Technique practitioner with over 25 years of experience in coaching and mentoring clients. She has the following degrees: Doctor of Ministry, Master of Science, Master of Divinity, and Bachelor of Arts. Additionally, she has a certificate in online teaching and learning and a postgraduate certificate in marriage and family therapy.

Connie Bynum is a health and wellness mentor, Young Living Essential Oils distributor, and former licensed massage therapist with over 20 years of experience in the field of natural health. She is well known for her expansive knowledge of essential oils and often speaks at workshops throughout the United States.

Connie and Kathy are sisters who love collaboration.

# Endnotes

[1] Bronzite, 2019.
[2] Alderson, 2019.
[3] Algoe, Kurtz, & Grewen, 2017.
[4] Schneiderman, Zagoory-Sharon, Leckman, & Feldman, 2012
[5] Wudarczyk, Earp, Guastella, & Savulescu, 2013.
[6] Wudarczyk et al., 2013.
[7] Wudarczyk et al., 2013.
[8] Gottman, 2019.
[9] Gottman, 2019.
[10] Mojay, 1999.
[11] Gottman, 2002.
[12] Helm, 2017.
[13] Helm, 2017.
[14] Seal et al., 2015.
[15] Higgins, 2016.
[16] Bloom & Bloom, 2016.
[17] McKenna, 2017.
[18] Lee, 1999.
[19] Battaglia, 2019.
[20] Loughran & Bull, 2001.
[21] Zeck, 2008.
[22] Institute, 2018.
[23] Hendrick, Hendrick, & Zacchilli, 2011.
[24] Hendrick & Hendrick, 2006.
[25] Hendrick et al., 2011.
[26] Hendrick & Hendrick, 2006.
[27] Hendrick et al., 2011.
[28] Bellows, 2018.
[29] Dashnaw, 2018.
[30] Dashnaw, 2018.
[31] Dashnaw, 2018.
[32] Dashnaw, 2018.

[33] Dashnaw, 2018.
[34] Gottman, 2019.
[35] Zeck, 2008.
[36] Poivre & Duez, 2017.
[37] Davis, 1991.
[38] Mojay, 1999.
[39] Zeck, 2008.
[40] "What % of your life," 2019.
[41] Guinness, 2015.
[42] Floyd, Hess, Miczo, Halone, Mikkelson, & Tusing, 2009.
[43] Floyd et al., 2009.
[44] Seppala, 2012.
[45] Floyd et al., 2009.
[46] Gulledge, Gulledge, & Stahmann, 2003.
[47] Gulledge et al., 2003.
[48] Whitbourne, 2014.
[49] Cohen, 2016.
[50] Pauley, Hesse, & Mikkelson, 2014.
[51] Zeck, 2008.
[52] Elmore, 2019.
[53] Bonior, 2018.
[54] Lewicki & Wiethoff, 2000.
[55] Lewicki & Wiethoff, 2000.
[56] Khalifian & Barry, 2016.
[57] Campbell, Boldry, Simpson, & Rubin, 2010.
[58] Josephs, 2018.
[59] Josephs, 2018.
[60] Josephs, 2018.
[61] Gottman, 2011.
[62] Theiss & Solomon, 2006.
[63] Khalifian & Barry, 2016.
[64] Lewicki & Wiethoff, 2000.
[65] Murray et al., 2006.
[66] Campbell et al., 2010.
[67] Lewicki & Wiethoff, 2000.

68 Bonior, 2018.
69 Zeck, 2008.
70 Fischer-Rizzi, 1991.
71 Young Living, 2019.
72 Young Living, 2019.
73 Young Living, 2019.
74 Ackerman, 2019.
75 Bockarova, 2018.
76 Papp, Goeke-Morey, & Cummings, 2013.
77 Yoo, Bartle-Haring, Day, & Gangamma, 2014.
78 Lenbuck, 2018.
79 Yoo et al., 2014.
80 Meston, & Stanton, 2019.
81 Papp et al, 2013.
82 Papp et al, 2013.
83 Cohen, 2019.
84 Gaspard, 2016.
85 Gaspard, 2016.
86 Arangua, 2018.
87 Seppala, 2012.
88 Battaglia, 2018.
89 Battaglia, 2018.
90 Davis, 1991.
91 Loughran, & Bull, 2001.
92 Mojay, 1999.
93 Frank & Brandstätter, 2002.
94 Kessler, 2015.
95 Weigel & Ballard-Reisch, 2014.
96 Frank & Brandstätter, 2002.
97 Frank & Brandstätter, 2002.
98 Frank & Brandstätter, 2002.
99 Guilbault & Philippe, 2017.
100 Gottman & Gottman, 2019.
101 Kessler, 2015.
102 Kessler, 2015.
103 Weigel & Ballard-Reisch, 2014.

[104] Weigel & Ballard-Reisch, 2014.
[105] Weigel & Ballard-Reisch, 2014.
[106] Battaglia, 2018.
[107] Battaglia, 2018.
[108] Loughran & Bull, 1991.
[109] Worwood, 1999.
[110] Gottman & Gottman, 2019.
[111] Seppala, 2012.
[112] Gottman & Gottman, 2019.
[113] Gottman & Gottman, 2019.
[114] Lavner, Karney, & Bradbury, 2016.
[115] See quote at the beginning of chapter 8.
[116] Gottman & Gottman, 2019.
[117] Uwom-Ajaegbu, Ajike, Fadolapo, & Ajaegbu, 2015.
[118] Uwom-Ajaegbu, Ajike, Fadolapo, & Ajaegbu, 2015.
[119] Battaglia, 2018.
[120] Mojay, 1999.
[121] Zeck, 2008.
[122] Emery, 2017.
[123] Rose, Anderson, Miller, Marks, Hatch, & Card, 2018.
[124] Orathinkal & Vansteenwegen, 2006.
[125] Fincham & Beach, 2002.
[126] Miller & Worthington, 2010.
[127] Russell, Baker, McNulty, & Overall, 2018.
[128] McNulty & Russell, 2016.
[129] Fife, Weeks, & Stellberg-Filbert, 2013.
[130] Worthington, 2010.
[131] Parrott & Parrott, 2017.
[132] Uglow, 2019.
[133] Uglow, 2019.
[134] Mojay, 1999.
[135] Loughran & Bull, 1991.
[136] Zeck, 2008.
[137] U.S. Census Bureau, 2006.
[138] Stepler, 2017.

[139] Stepler, 2017.
[140] Brown, 2019.
[141] Brown, 2019.
[142] Brown, 2019.
[143] Gottman, 1994.
[144] Gottman, 1994.
[145] Johnson, Stanley, Glenn, Amato, Nock, Markman, & Dion, 2002.
[146] Gottman & Silver, 2000.
[147] Gottman & Silver, 2000.

www.ingramcontent.com/pod-product-compliance
Lightning Source LLC
Chambersburg PA
CBHW030703220526
45463CB00005B/1881